The Complete
ULCERATIVE COLITIS COOKBOOK

Delectable Step-By-Step Recipes to Manage Symptoms, Improve Digestive System and Reduce Inflammation

Nancy Rios

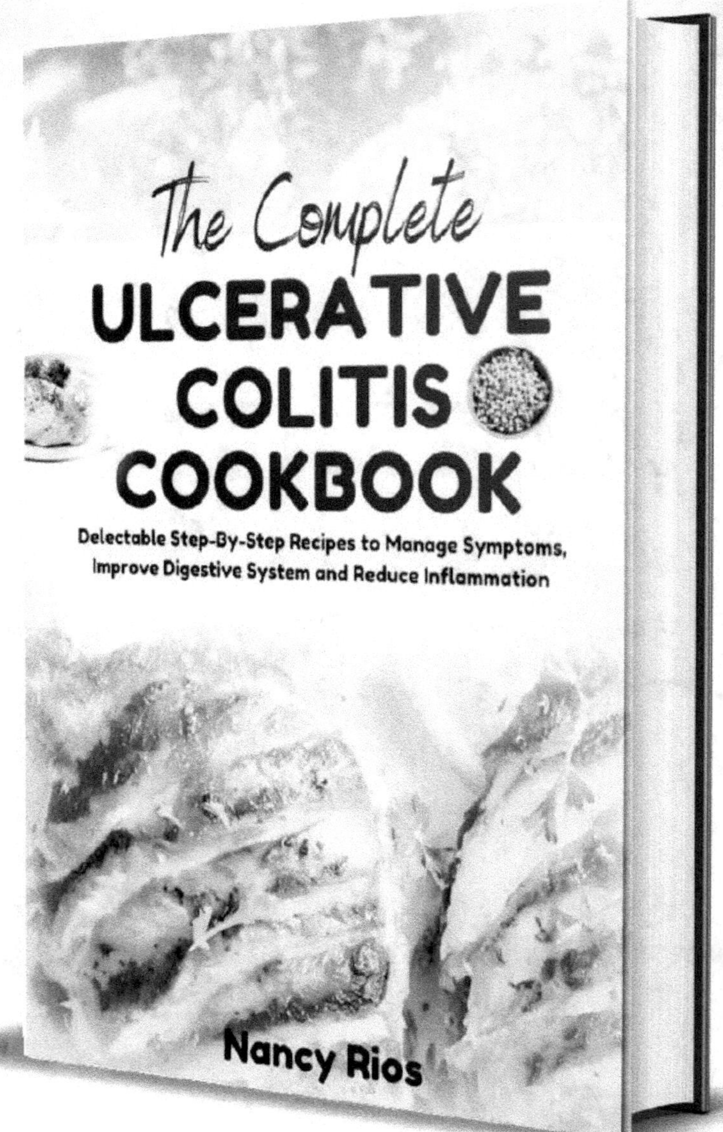
The Complete
ULCERATIVE
COLITIS
COOKBOOK
Delectable Step-By-Step Recipes to Manage Symptoms,
Improve Digestive System and Reduce Inflammation
Nancy Rios

Copyright © 2024 Nancy Rios

DEDICATION

To all those who face the daily challenges of living with ulcerative colitis: this book is dedicated to you. Your resilience and strength in managing this condition are truly inspiring. It is with you in mind that every recipe, tip, and piece of advice has been crafted. Your journey toward better health and comfort through food deserves every bit of attention and care.

To the healthcare professionals and nutritionists who provide invaluable support and guidance—thank you for your dedication and expertise. Your commitment to improving lives through knowledge and compassion has been a guiding light in creating this cookbook.

And to my loved ones, whose unwavering support and encouragement have been my foundation throughout this project—your belief in me has made this book possible.

This cookbook is a celebration of hope, healing, and the simple joy of nourishing your body with food that loves you back.

PREFACE

Welcome to **The Complete Ulcerative Colitis Cookbook**. This book is more than a collection of recipes; it's a practical guide designed to support your journey toward better health. If you're living with ulcerative colitis, you understand how crucial diet is to managing your symptoms and enhancing your quality of life. Through thoughtful meal planning and carefully chosen ingredients, this cookbook aims to provide relief and restore enjoyment in your daily meals.

Each recipe has been crafted with your well-being in mind, focusing on easy-to-digest, nutrient-rich foods that can help reduce inflammation and promote healing. Whether you're seeking comfort during a flare-up or looking for everyday meals that support your health, you'll find a variety of options tailored to your needs.

Thank you for choosing this book. I hope it becomes a valuable resource on your path to wellness and a source of inspiration for healthier, happier living.

ACKNOWLEDGEMENTS

Creating **The Complete Ulcerative Colitis Cookbook** has been a deeply rewarding journey, made possible by the support and contributions of many incredible individuals.

I extend my heartfelt thanks to the healthcare professionals and nutritionists whose expertise shaped this book, providing invaluable insights into managing ulcerative colitis through diet. To the patients and families who shared their stories and experiences, your courage and openness have been a source of inspiration. Special thanks to the recipe testers whose feedback ensured each dish is both delicious and suitable for those with sensitive digestive systems.

To my loved ones, your unwavering support and encouragement have been my anchor throughout this process. This book is dedicated to all who strive to find balance and joy in their lives despite the challenges of ulcerative colitis. Your trust and commitment to improving your health are what truly drive this work. Thank you.

Why This Book?

The Complete Ulcerative Colitis Cookbook stands out because it is meticulously designed to address the specific dietary needs of those living with ulcerative colitis. Unlike generic cookbooks, this book focuses on creating meals that are not only delicious but also gentle on your digestive system. Each recipe is crafted to minimize discomfort, reduce inflammation, and promote overall gut health.

This cookbook goes beyond mere recipe collections. It offers a comprehensive approach by incorporating essential information about ulcerative colitis, including its causes, symptoms, and risk factors. The book provides clear guidance on which foods to embrace and which to avoid, ensuring that you have practical strategies for managing your condition through diet.

Additionally, the meal plans and recipes are designed to fit seamlessly into your life, offering both convenience and nourishment.

Whether you're dealing with flare-ups or looking to maintain remission, the recipes here are tailored to provide comfort and support.

Choosing this book means choosing a resource that respects your needs and empowers you with the knowledge to make informed dietary choices. It's more than just a cookbook—it's a tool for improving your quality of life and embracing a healthier, more enjoyable way of eating.

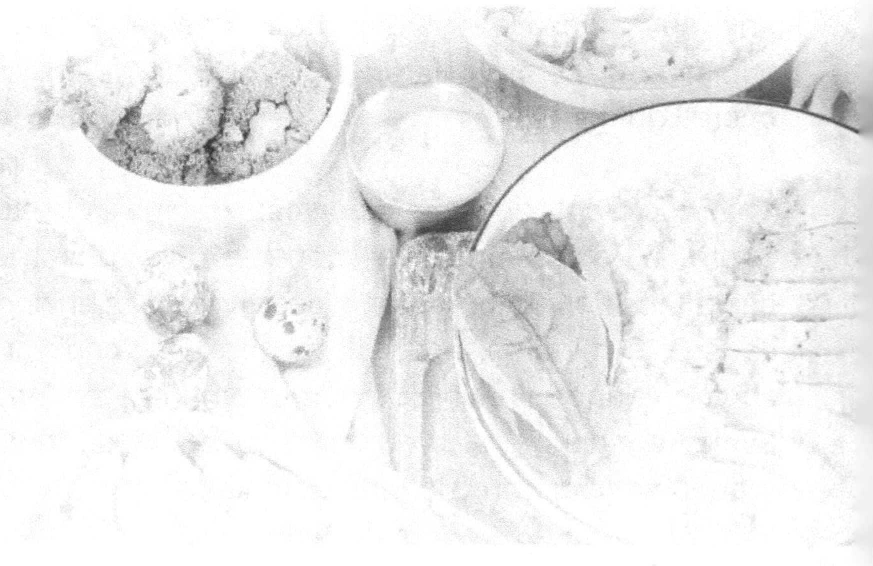

TABLE OF CONTENT

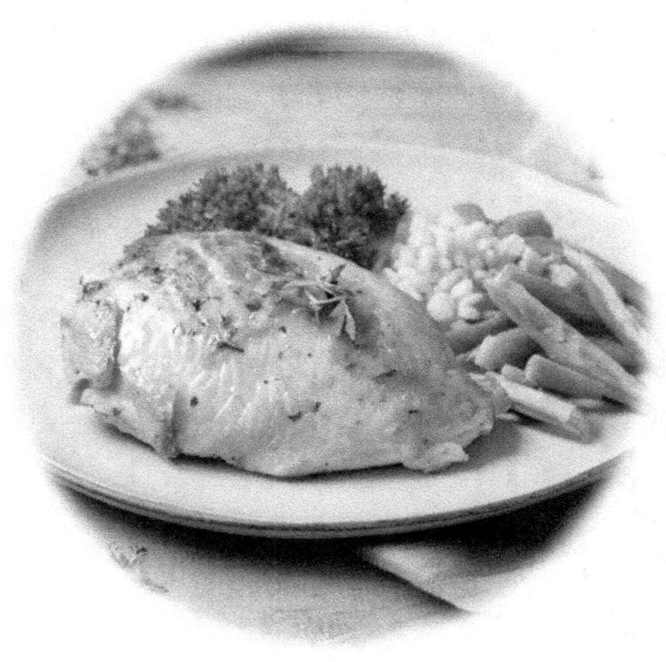

Introduction

Imagine waking up each day unsure of what lies ahead—not because of the hustle and bustle of life, but because of a chronic condition that has taken the driver's seat. Ulcerative colitis doesn't just affect your body; it affects your mind, your mood, and even your relationships.

The unpredictability of flare-ups, the discomfort, and the constant worry about what foods might trigger symptoms can be overwhelming.

For years, I watched a close friend struggle with this very reality.

Every meal was a gamble, every social gathering a source of anxiety.

The joy of eating was replaced by fear and uncertainty.

I saw the toll it took on her, not just physically, but emotionally.

She longed for normalcy, for a way to regain control over her life, and to enjoy food without the looming threat of pain.

That's when I knew something had to change. I delved deep into the world of nutrition and discovered that food could be a powerful tool— not just for survival, but for healing. I started experimenting with recipes, focusing on ingredients that were gentle on the gut, anti-inflammatory, and nourishing.

Slowly but surely, my friend began to notice a difference. Her flare-ups became less frequent, her energy levels improved, and she started to enjoy food again.

This cookbook is the result of that journey. It's not just a collection of recipes; it's a lifeline for those living with ulcerative colitis.

It's a guide to reclaiming your health and your happiness, one meal at a time. Each recipe has been carefully crafted to provide comfort, nutrition, and most importantly, to support your body in managing ulcerative colitis.

Whether you're newly diagnosed or have been living with ulcerative colitis for years, this book is for you.

It's for anyone who wants to take control of their health, who wants to find joy in food again, and who wants to live a life that isn't defined by their condition.

This isn't just a cookbook; it's a companion on your journey to wellness.

With The Complete Ulcerative Colitis Cookbook in your kitchen, you'll have the tools you need to make delicious, nourishing meals that work with your body, not against it. You'll find comfort in knowing that every recipe has been created with your well-being in mind.

And most importantly, you'll discover that living with ulcerative colitis doesn't mean giving up on the foods you love—it just means finding new ways to enjoy them.

So take the first step on your journey to better health. Let this book be your guide, and together, let's reclaim the joy of eating.

Understanding Ulcerative Colitis

What is Ulcerative Colitis?

Ulcerative colitis is a chronic inflammatory bowel disease that primarily affects the colon and rectum. It involves persistent inflammation and the development of small ulcers along the lining of the large intestine.

This inflammation leads to a range of symptoms, including abdominal pain, cramping, diarrhea, and an urgent need to use the bathroom. For many, these symptoms can be debilitating and disruptive to daily life.

The exact cause of ulcerative colitis remains unknown, but it is believed to result from an abnormal immune response where the body mistakenly attacks healthy tissues in the digestive tract.

Genetic factors, environmental triggers, and an overactive immune system are all thought to contribute to the disease's development.

Living with ulcerative colitis often requires careful management to control symptoms and prevent flare-ups. While medication and lifestyle changes are crucial, diet plays a pivotal role in managing the condition.

By choosing the right foods and avoiding potential triggers, individuals can reduce inflammation, promote healing, and improve their quality of life.

The Complete Ulcerative Colitis Cookbook provides a practical guide to navigating this complex condition, offering recipes and tips designed to support gut health and ease the symptoms of ulcerative colitis.

Causes of Ulcerative Colitis

Ulcerative colitis (UC) is a chronic inflammatory bowel disease that primarily affects the lining of the large intestine and rectum.

The exact cause of UC remains unclear, but research suggests a combination of factors contribute to its development.

Genetics play a significant role. Individuals with a family history of UC or other inflammatory bowel diseases are more likely to develop the condition.

Specific genetic mutations have been linked to a higher risk, though not everyone with these mutations will develop UC.

Immune system dysfunction is another critical factor. In UC, the immune system mistakenly attacks the healthy cells in the colon, causing inflammation and ulcers.

This abnormal immune response may be triggered by environmental factors, such as bacterial or viral infections.

Environmental factors can also influence the onset of UC. Diet, stress, and exposure to certain medications or pollutants may increase susceptibility.

While these factors don't directly cause UC, they can exacerbate symptoms or trigger flare-ups in those predisposed to the disease.

Understanding the causes of UC is vital in managing the condition.

By recognizing the genetic, immune, and environmental factors at play, individuals can make informed decisions about their diet and lifestyle to better manage their health.

Symptoms and Diagnosis

The symptoms can vary in intensity, but they often include persistent diarrhea, abdominal pain, and cramping.

Other common signs include blood or pus in the stool, an urgent need to have a bowel movement, and unintended weight loss.

Fatigue and fever may also occur, reflecting the body's inflammatory response.

The unpredictability of symptoms, which can range from mild to severe, makes ulcerative colitis particularly challenging.

Flare-ups can disrupt daily life, leading to discomfort, stress, and anxiety. Understanding these symptoms is crucial for managing the condition effectively.

Diagnosing ulcerative colitis typically involves a combination of medical history, physical examination, and diagnostic tests.

Blood tests can detect anemia or signs of inflammation, while stool samples may reveal infections or bleeding.

However, the definitive diagnosis often requires endoscopic procedures, such as colonoscopy or sigmoidoscopy, where a specialist visually examines the colon and takes tissue biopsies.

Early diagnosis and intervention are key to managing ulcerative colitis and preventing complications.

By understanding the symptoms and seeking prompt medical care, individuals can better control the condition and improve their quality of life.

Risk Factors

Ulcerative colitis is a chronic inflammatory bowel disease that affects the colon and rectum, and while its exact cause remains unclear, several risk factors can increase the likelihood of developing the condition.

Genetics play a significant role, with a higher risk observed in individuals who have a family history of ulcerative colitis or other autoimmune diseases.

Environmental factors, such as living in developed countries or urban areas, have also been linked to a greater prevalence of the disease, possibly due to dietary habits, pollution, or other lifestyle factors.

Age is another important factor, as ulcerative colitis is most commonly diagnosed in people under the age of 30, though it can occur at any age. Additionally, certain medications, particularly nonsteroidal anti-inflammatory drugs (NSAIDs), have been associated with an increased risk of triggering or exacerbating symptoms.

Finally, smoking and stress, while not direct causes, can influence the severity and frequency of flare-ups in those already diagnosed.

Understanding these risk factors is crucial for both prevention and effective management, as it empowers individuals to make informed choices that can minimize their risk and improve their quality of life.

The Role of Diet in Managing Ulcerative Colitis

Benefits of Following a Specialized Diet

Following a specialized diet for ulcerative colitis is essential for managing symptoms and improving quality of life. By carefully selecting foods that are gentle on the digestive system, you can significantly reduce the frequency and severity of flare-ups.

A well-planned diet helps minimize inflammation, promotes healing of the gut lining, and ensures that you receive the necessary nutrients to support overall health.

A specialized diet tailored to ulcerative colitis is more than just a meal plan—it's a proactive approach to managing the condition.

It empowers you to take control of your health by focusing on foods that are easy to digest and avoiding those that could trigger symptoms.

By doing so, you can experience fewer disruptions in your daily life, maintain better energy levels, and enjoy meals without fear of discomfort.

In addition to managing symptoms, a targeted diet also plays a crucial role in preventing complications associated with ulcerative colitis, such as nutrient deficiencies and weight loss.

With the right dietary choices, you can enhance your well-being, support your body's natural healing processes, and live a more comfortable, fulfilling life despite the challenges of ulcerative colitis.

Foods to Eat and Avoid

When managing ulcerative colitis, your food choices are crucial in minimizing symptoms and promoting gut health.

While there's no one-size-fits-all diet, certain foods are generally beneficial, while others may exacerbate symptoms.

Foods to Eat: Focus on nourishing, easy-to-digest options. Lean proteins like chicken, turkey, and fish are excellent choices, providing the body with essential nutrients without causing irritation.

Incorporate cooked vegetables such as carrots, zucchini, and spinach, which are gentle on the digestive system. Low-fiber fruits like bananas, applesauce, and melons are also well-tolerated. Whole grains like white rice and oatmeal can provide energy without straining the gut.

Additionally, probiotic-rich foods like yogurt can support a healthy balance of gut bacteria.

Foods to Avoid: Certain foods can trigger flare-ups or worsen symptoms. High-fiber foods like raw vegetables, whole nuts, and seeds can be harsh on the digestive tract and are best avoided.

Spicy foods, caffeine, and alcohol can irritate the gut lining, leading to discomfort.

Fatty and fried foods are also problematic, as they can be difficult to digest and may increase inflammation. Additionally, dairy products might need to be limited if lactose intolerance is a concern.

By making informed dietary choices, you can better manage your symptoms and improve your quality of life with ulcerative colitis.

How to Use This Cookbook

Navigating Recipes and Meal Plans

Creating a meal plan that supports your health while managing ulcerative colitis can seem daunting, but with The Complete Ulcerative Colitis Cookbook, it becomes a more straightforward process.

This cookbook is designed to make your journey smoother by providing clear, easy-to-follow recipes tailored to your unique needs.

Each recipe is carefully crafted to prioritize gentle, gut-friendly ingredients that help minimize inflammation and avoid triggering symptoms.

Meal planning is about more than just what to eat; it's about making informed choices that suit your lifestyle and nutritional requirements.

In this book, you'll find recipes categorized by meal type, making it simple to mix and match dishes throughout the week.

Whether you need a quick breakfast that's easy on the stomach or a hearty dinner that won't cause discomfort, the options are plentiful and varied.

Each recipe is accompanied by tips on how to modify it based on your current condition, whether you're in remission or experiencing a flare-up. The book also includes practical advice on portion control, food preparation, and storing leftovers, ensuring that your meal plan is not only nourishing but also sustainable in the long term.

Tips for Cooking and Meal Planning

Cooking and meal planning for ulcerative colitis requires thoughtful preparation to ensure that every dish is not only delicious but also gentle on your digestive system.

Begin by choosing simple, whole foods that are easy to digest and low in irritants. Focus on ingredients like lean proteins, cooked vegetables, and easily digestible grains.

Batch cooking is a powerful strategy. Prepare larger portions of meals and store them in single-serving containers. This way, you'll always have a safe, ready-to-eat option on hand, reducing the stress of daily meal decisions.

When cooking, use methods like steaming, boiling, or baking, which are less likely to cause irritation.

Avoid deep frying or grilling at high temperatures, as these can exacerbate symptoms.

Plan your meals around what your body tolerates best, keeping a food diary to track any triggers.

Incorporate a variety of textures and flavors to keep meals enjoyable, and don't shy away from experimenting with herbs that add flavor without causing flare-ups.

Lastly, stay hydrated with plenty of water and gentle herbal teas. By being proactive and organized in your meal planning, you'll find it easier to manage your symptoms while still enjoying a varied and satisfying diet.

Chapter 1: Breakfast

1. Creamy Oatmeal with Banana

Ingredients:

1 cup rolled oats

2 cups water

1 ripe banana, sliced

1 tablespoon honey (optional)

1/2 teaspoon cinnamon

Pinch of salt

Instructions:

In a medium saucepan, combine the oats, water, and salt. Bring to a boil.

Reduce heat and simmer for 5-7 minutes, stirring occasionally, until the oats are soft and the mixture has thickened.

Remove from heat and stir in the sliced banana, honey (if using), and cinnamon.

Let it sit for a few minutes before serving.

Cooking Time: 10 minutes

2. Scrambled Eggs with Spinach

Ingredients:

2 large eggs

1 cup fresh spinach, chopped

1 tablespoon olive oil

Salt and pepper to taste

Instructions:

Heat the olive oil in a non-stick skillet over medium heat.

Add the spinach and cook until wilted, about 1-2 minutes.

In a bowl, whisk the eggs with a pinch of salt and pepper.

Pour the eggs into the skillet and cook, stirring gently, until they are just set.

Serve immediately.

Cooking Time: 5 minutes

3. Smoothie with Blueberries and Yogurt

Ingredients:

1/2 cup fresh or frozen blueberries

1 cup plain yogurt (or a dairy-free alternative)

1/2 banana

1/2 cup water or almond milk

1 teaspoon honey (optional)

Instructions:

Place all ingredients into a blender.

Blend until smooth.

Pour into a glass and serve immediately.

Cooking Time: 5 minutes

4. Apple Cinnamon Quinoa Porridge

Ingredients:

1/2 cup quinoa, rinsed

1 cup water

1/2 apple, peeled and diced

1/2 teaspoon cinnamon

1 tablespoon maple syrup (optional)

Pinch of salt

Instructions:

In a saucepan, combine quinoa, water, and salt. Bring to a boil.

Reduce heat, cover, and simmer for 15 minutes, or until quinoa is cooked.

Stir in the diced apple, cinnamon, and maple syrup (if using).

Cook for an additional 2-3 minutes, until apples are tender.

Cooking Time: 20 minutes

5. Soft-Baked Sweet Potato Hash

Ingredients:

1 large sweet potato, peeled and diced

1 tablespoon olive oil

1/2 teaspoon dried thyme

Salt and pepper to taste

Instructions:

Preheat the oven to 400°F (200°C).

Toss the sweet potato cubes with olive oil, thyme, salt, and pepper.

Spread the sweet potato on a baking sheet in a single layer.

Bake for 20-25 minutes, or until tender, stirring halfway through.

Cooking Time: 25 minutes

6. Pumpkin Spice Chia Pudding

Ingredients:

1/4 cup chia seeds

1 cup almond milk

1/4 cup pumpkin puree

1 tablespoon maple syrup

1/2 teaspoon pumpkin pie spice

Instructions:

In a bowl, combine chia seeds, almond milk, pumpkin puree, maple syrup, and pumpkin pie spice.

Stir well and refrigerate for at least 4 hours or overnight.

Stir before serving.

Cooking Time: 4 hours (chilling time)

7. Overnight Oats with Almond Milk

Ingredients:

1/2 cup rolled oats

1/2 cup almond milk

1/2 tablespoon chia seeds

1 tablespoon honey or maple syrup (optional)

Fresh fruit for topping

Instructions:

In a jar or container, combine oats, almond milk, chia seeds, and sweetener (if using).

Stir well, cover, and refrigerate overnight.

In the morning, stir and top with fresh fruit before serving.

Cooking Time: 5 minutes (plus overnight refrigeration)

8. Cottage Cheese and Berries Parfait

Ingredients:

1 cup cottage cheese

1/2 cup fresh berries (e.g., blueberries, strawberries)

1 tablespoon honey (optional)

1/4 cup granola (optional)

Instructions:

In a bowl or glass, layer cottage cheese with berries.

Drizzle with honey (if using).

Top with granola, if desired.

Cooking Time: 5 minutes

9. Simple Rice Porridge

Ingredients:

1/2 cup white rice

1 cup water

1/2 cup almond milk

1 tablespoon honey (optional)

Pinch of salt

Instructions:

In a saucepan, bring rice and water to a boil.

Reduce heat, cover, and simmer for 15 minutes, or until rice is tender.

Stir in almond milk, honey (if using), and salt.

Cook for an additional 5 minutes until creamy.

Cooking Time: 20 minutes

10. Herbal Tea with Ginger and Lemon

Ingredients:

1 cup water

1 ginger slice (about 1 inch)

1 herbal tea bag (e.g., chamomile or peppermint)

1 lemon slice

Honey (optional)

Instructions:

Boil the water and add the ginger slice.

Let it simmer for 5 minutes.

Remove from heat and steep the tea bag for 3-5 minutes. Remove the tea bag, ginger slice, and add the lemon slice.

Sweeten with honey if desired.

Cooking Time: 10 minutes

11. Chicken Bone Broth

Ingredients:

2 pounds chicken bones (from rotisserie or raw)

1 onion, quartered

2 carrots, chopped

2 celery stalks, chopped

3 garlic cloves, peeled

2 bay leaves

1 teaspoon black peppercorns

1 tablespoon apple cider vinegar

8 cups water

Instructions:

Preheat your oven to 400°F (200°C). Spread the chicken bones on a baking sheet and roast for 30 minutes, turning halfway through.

Transfer the roasted bones to a large pot or slow cooker. Add the onion, carrots, celery, garlic, bay leaves, and peppercorns.

Pour in the water and apple cider vinegar. Bring to a boil, then reduce to a simmer.

Simmer for 4-6 hours, skimming off any foam that rises to the surface.

Strain the broth through a fine-mesh sieve. Discard the solids and let the broth cool.

Store in the refrigerator for up to 5 days or freeze for up to 3 months.

Cooking Time: 4-6 hours

12. Carrot and Ginger Soup

Ingredients:

1 tablespoon olive oil

1 onion, chopped

4 cups carrots, peeled and sliced

1 tablespoon fresh ginger, grated

4 cups vegetable broth (low-sodium)

Salt and pepper to taste

1/2 cup coconut milk (optional)

Instructions:

Heat olive oil in a large pot over medium heat. Add the onion and cook until softened, about 5 minutes.

Add the carrots and ginger, cooking for another 5 minutes.

Pour in the vegetable broth and bring to a boil. Reduce heat and simmer until carrots are tender, about 20 minutes.

Use an immersion blender to puree the soup until smooth. Alternatively, carefully transfer to a blender in batches.

Stir in coconut milk if using and season with salt and pepper.

Cooking Time: 30 minutes

13. Creamy Butternut Squash Soup

Ingredients:

1 tablespoon olive oil

1 onion, chopped

1 medium butternut squash, peeled and cubed

2 cloves garlic, minced

4 cups vegetable broth (low-sodium)

1/2 teaspoon ground nutmeg

Salt and pepper to taste

1/2 cup plain yogurt (optional)

Instructions:

Heat olive oil in a large pot over medium heat. Add onion and cook until translucent, about 5 minutes.

Add the butternut squash and garlic, cooking for another 5 minutes.

Pour in the vegetable broth and bring to a boil. Reduce heat and simmer until squash is tender, about 20 minutes.

Use an immersion blender to puree the soup until smooth. Alternatively, transfer to a blender in batches.

Stir in yogurt if using and season with nutmeg, salt, and pepper.

Cooking Time: 30 minutes

14. Simple Chicken and Rice Soup

Ingredients:

1 tablespoon olive oil

1 onion, chopped

2 carrots, sliced

2 celery stalks, sliced

1 cup cooked chicken, shredded

1/2 cup rice (white or brown)

4 cups chicken broth (low-sodium)

Salt and pepper to taste

Instructions:

Heat olive oil in a large pot over medium heat. Add onion, carrots, and celery, cooking until softened, about 5 minutes.

Add chicken broth and bring to a boil. Stir in the rice and cook for 10 minutes.

Add the cooked chicken and simmer for another 5 minutes.

Season with salt and pepper to taste.

Cooking Time: 20 minutes

15. Sweet Potato and Leek Soup

Ingredients:

1 tablespoon olive oil

1 leek, white and light green parts only, sliced

2 sweet potatoes, peeled and cubed

4 cups vegetable broth (low-sodium)

1 teaspoon dried thyme

Salt and pepper to taste

Instructions:

Heat olive oil in a large pot over medium heat. Add leeks and cook until softened, about 5 minutes.

Add sweet potatoes and cook for another 5 minutes.

Pour in the vegetable broth and bring to a boil. Reduce heat and simmer until sweet potatoes are tender, about 20 minutes.

Use an immersion blender to puree the soup until smooth. Alternatively, transfer to a blender in batches.

Season with thyme, salt, and pepper.

Cooking Time: 30 minutes

16. Mild Tomato Soup

Ingredients:

1 tablespoon olive oil

1 onion, chopped

2 garlic cloves, minced

4 cups canned tomatoes (diced or whole, no added salt)

2 cups vegetable broth (low-sodium)

1 teaspoon dried basil

Salt and pepper to taste

Instructions:

Heat olive oil in a large pot over medium heat. Add onion and garlic, cooking until softened, about 5 minutes.

Add tomatoes and vegetable broth, bring to a boil.

Reduce heat and simmer for 15 minutes.

Use an immersion blender to puree the soup until smooth. Alternatively, transfer to a blender in batches.

Stir in basil and season with salt and pepper.

Cooking Time: 20 minutes

17. Pureed Cauliflower Soup

Ingredients:

1 tablespoon olive oil

1 onion, chopped

1 head cauliflower, cut into florets

4 cups vegetable broth (low-sodium)

1/2 teaspoon garlic powder

Salt and pepper to taste

Instructions:

Heat olive oil in a large pot over medium heat. Add onion and cook until softened, about 5 minutes.

Add cauliflower and cook for another 5 minutes.

Pour in vegetable broth and bring to a boil. Reduce heat and simmer until cauliflower is tender, about 15 minutes.

Use an immersion blender to puree the soup until smooth. Alternatively, transfer to a blender in batches.

Season with garlic powder, salt, and pepper.

Cooking Time: 20 minutes

18. Zucchini and Basil Soup

Ingredients:

1 tablespoon olive oil

1 onion, chopped

4 zucchinis, sliced

4 cups vegetable broth (low-sodium)

1/2 cup fresh basil leaves

Salt and pepper to taste

Instructions:

Heat olive oil in a large pot over medium heat. Add onion and cook until softened, about 5 minutes.

Add zucchini and cook for another 5 minutes.

Pour in vegetable broth and bring to a boil. Reduce heat and simmer until zucchini is tender, about 15 minutes.

Add basil and use an immersion blender to puree the soup until smooth. Alternatively, transfer to a blender in batches.

Season with salt and pepper.

Cooking Time: 20 minutes

19. Healing Miso Broth

Ingredients:

4 cups water

1/4 cup miso paste (white or yellow)

1 tablespoon grated ginger

1 small carrot, sliced

1 green onion, sliced

Instructions:

Heat water in a pot over medium heat. Add ginger and carrot, simmer for 10 minutes.

Reduce heat to low and whisk in miso paste until fully dissolved.

Add green onion and simmer for an additional 5 minutes.

Serve warm.

Cooking Time: 15 minutes

20. Spinach and Potato Soup

Ingredients:

1 tablespoon olive oil

1 onion, chopped

2 potatoes, peeled and cubed

4 cups vegetable broth (low-sodium)

2 cups fresh spinach

Salt and pepper to taste

Instructions:

Heat olive oil in a large pot over medium heat. Add onion and cook until softened, about 5 minutes.

Add potatoes and cook for another 5 minutes.

Pour in vegetable broth and bring to a boil. Reduce heat and simmer until potatoes are tender, about 15 minutes.

Stir in spinach and cook until wilted, about 3 minutes.

Use an immersion blender to puree the soup until smooth. Alternatively, transfer to a blender in batches.

Season with salt and pepper.

Cooking Time: 20 minutes

21. Baked Chicken Breast with Herbs

Ingredients:

4 boneless, skinless chicken breasts

2 tablespoons olive oil

1 teaspoon dried thyme

1 teaspoon dried rosemary

1 teaspoon dried oregano

Salt and pepper to taste

2 cloves garlic, minced (optional)

Instructions:

Preheat the oven to 375°F (190°C).

Rub each chicken breast with olive oil and sprinkle with thyme, rosemary, oregano, salt, and pepper. Add minced garlic if desired.

Place the chicken breasts in a baking dish.

Bake for 25-30 minutes, or until the internal temperature reaches 165°F (74°C) and the chicken is cooked through.

Let the chicken rest for 5 minutes before slicing.

Cooking Time: 25-30 minutes

22. Steamed Fish with Lemon and Dill

Ingredients:

4 fish fillets (such as cod or tilapia)

1 lemon, thinly sliced

2 tablespoons fresh dill, chopped (or 1 tablespoon dried dill)

Salt and pepper to taste

1 tablespoon olive oil

Instructions:

Place a steamer basket over a pot of simmering water.

Season the fish fillets with salt, pepper, and dill.

Place lemon slices on top of the fish.

Place the fish in the steamer basket.

Cover and steam for 8-10 minutes, or until the fish is opaque and flakes easily with a fork.

Drizzle with olive oil before serving.

Cooking Time: 8-10 minutes

23. Quinoa Salad with Cucumbers and Herbs

Ingredients:

1 cup quinoa

2 cups water or low-sodium vegetable broth

1 cup cucumber, diced

1/4 cup fresh parsley, chopped

1/4 cup fresh mint, chopped

2 tablespoons olive oil

1 tablespoon lemon juice

Salt and pepper to taste

Instructions:

Rinse the quinoa under cold water.

In a medium pot, bring water or broth to a boil. Add quinoa, reduce heat, and simmer for 15 minutes, or until quinoa is tender and liquid is absorbed.

Fluff quinoa with a fork and let it cool to room temperature.

In a large bowl, combine quinoa, cucumber, parsley, and mint.

Whisk together olive oil, lemon juice, salt, and pepper. Pour over the salad and toss to combine.

Cooking Time: 15 minutes (plus cooling time)

24. Turkey and Sweet Potato Skillet

Ingredients:

1 lb (450g) ground turkey

2 medium sweet potatoes, peeled and diced

1 tablespoon olive oil

1 teaspoon ground cumin

1 teaspoon paprika

1/2 teaspoon garlic powder

Salt and pepper to taste

1 cup spinach, chopped (optional)

Instructions:

Heat olive oil in a large skillet over medium heat.

Add ground turkey and cook until browned, breaking it up with a spoon.

Add diced sweet potatoes, cumin, paprika, garlic powder, salt, and pepper. Stir well.

Cover and cook for 15-20 minutes, or until sweet potatoes are tender.

Stir in spinach, if using, and cook for an additional 2-3 minutes, until wilted.

Cooking Time: 15-20 minutes

25. Mild Vegetable Stir-Fry

Ingredients:

2 tablespoons olive oil

1 cup carrots, thinly sliced

1 cup zucchini, sliced

1 cup bell peppers, sliced

1 cup broccoli florets

2 tablespoons low-sodium soy sauce (optional)

1 tablespoon ginger, minced

Salt to taste

Instructions:

Heat olive oil in a large skillet or wok over medium heat.

Add ginger and cook for 1 minute.

Add carrots, zucchini, bell peppers, and broccoli. Stir-fry for 5-7 minutes, or until vegetables are tender-crisp.

If using, add soy sauce and stir well. Cook for an additional 2 minutes.

Cooking Time: 7-10 minutes

26. Baked Salmon with Dill Sauce

Ingredients:

4 salmon fillets

2 tablespoons olive oil

1 tablespoon fresh dill, chopped (or 1 teaspoon dried dill)

1 tablespoon lemon juice

Salt and pepper to taste

1/2 cup plain Greek yogurt (for the sauce)

Instructions:

Preheat the oven to 375°F (190°C).

Rub salmon fillets with olive oil, dill, lemon juice, salt, and pepper.

Place the salmon in a baking dish.

Bake for 15-20 minutes, or until the fish flakes easily with a fork.

For the dill sauce, mix Greek yogurt with additional dill and a splash of lemon juice.

Cooking Time: 15-20 minutes

27. Stuffed Bell Peppers with Rice

Ingredients:

4 large bell peppers, tops cut off and seeds removed

1 cup cooked rice

1/2 lb (225g) ground beef or turkey

1 cup tomato sauce

1/2 cup chopped onion

1 teaspoon dried oregano

Salt and pepper to taste

Instructions:

Preheat the oven to 375°F (190°C).

Cook ground beef or turkey with onions until browned. Drain any excess fat.

In a bowl, combine cooked rice, meat mixture, tomato sauce, oregano, salt, and pepper.

Stuff the bell peppers with the mixture.

Place the stuffed peppers in a baking dish and cover with foil.

Bake for 30-35 minutes, or until peppers are tender.

Cooking Time: 30-35 minutes

28. Chicken and Carrot Stew

Ingredients:

1 lb (450g) boneless, skinless chicken thighs, cut into pieces

4 carrots, peeled and sliced

1 tablespoon olive oil

1 cup low-sodium chicken broth

1 teaspoon dried thyme

Salt and pepper to taste

Instructions:

Heat olive oil in a large pot over medium heat.

Add chicken pieces and cook until browned.

Add carrots, chicken broth, thyme, salt, and pepper. Bring to a simmer.

Cover and cook for 20-25 minutes, or until chicken is cooked through and carrots are tender.

Cooking Time: 20-25 minutes

29. Soft-Cooked Pasta with Olive Oil and Herbs

Ingredients:

8 oz (225g) pasta (such as penne or fusilli)

2 tablespoons olive oil

1 tablespoon fresh basil, chopped

1 tablespoon fresh parsley, chopped

Salt to taste

Instructions:

Cook pasta according to package instructions until very soft.

Drain and return to the pot.

Stir in olive oil, basil, parsley, and salt.

Cook over low heat for 2-3 minutes to combine flavors.

Cooking Time: 8-10 minutes

30. Simple Ground Turkey and Spinach

Ingredients:

1 lb (450g) ground turkey

2 cups fresh spinach, chopped

1 tablespoon olive oil

1 teaspoon garlic powder

Salt and pepper to taste

Instructions:

Heat olive oil in a skillet over medium heat.

Add ground turkey and cook until browned, breaking it up with a spoon.

Stir in garlic powder, salt, and pepper.

Add spinach and cook for 2-3 minutes, or until wilted.

Cooking Time: 10-12 minutes

31. Apple Slices with Almond Butter

Ingredients:

1 large apple (any variety)

2 tablespoons almond butter

A sprinkle of cinnamon (optional)

Instructions:

Core and slice the apple into thin wedges.

Spread almond butter evenly on each apple slice.

Sprinkle with a pinch of cinnamon if desired.

Serve immediately or pack in an airtight container for a portable snack.

Cooking Time: None (prep time: 5 minutes)

32. Soft-Baked Oatmeal Cookies

Ingredients:

1 cup rolled oats

1/2 cup mashed banana (about 1 large banana)

1/4 cup almond flour

1/4 cup honey or maple syrup

1/2 teaspoon vanilla extract

1/4 teaspoon baking soda

A pinch of salt

Instructions:

Preheat oven to 350°F (175°C) and line a baking sheet with parchment paper.

In a bowl, mix together the oats, almond flour, baking soda, and salt.

In another bowl, combine the mashed banana, honey, and vanilla extract.

Add the wet ingredients to the dry ingredients and mix until well combined.

Scoop tablespoons of the mixture onto the prepared baking sheet, flattening slightly.

Bake for 10-12 minutes, or until edges are golden brown.

Allow cookies to cool on a wire rack before serving.

Cooking Time: 10-12 minutes

33. Carrot Sticks with Hummus

Ingredients:

3 large carrots

1/2 cup plain hummus

Instructions:

Peel the carrots and cut them into sticks.

Serve the carrot sticks with hummus for dipping.

Cooking Time: None (prep time: 5 minutes)

34. Rice Cakes with Avocado

Ingredients:

2 plain rice cakes

1 ripe avocado

Salt and pepper to taste

A squeeze of lemon juice (optional)

Instructions:

Peel and mash the avocado in a bowl.

Season with salt, pepper, and a squeeze of lemon juice if desired.

Spread the mashed avocado evenly over the rice cakes.

Serve immediately.

Cooking Time: None (prep time: 5 minutes)

35. Yogurt with Honey and Blueberries

Ingredients:

1 cup plain yogurt (such as Greek or regular)

1 tablespoon honey

1/4 cup fresh blueberries

Instructions:

Spoon the yogurt into a bowl.

Drizzle honey over the yogurt.

Top with fresh blueberries.

Serve immediately.

Cooking Time: None (prep time: 5 minutes)

36. Smoothie Popsicles

Ingredients:

1 cup frozen mixed berries

1/2 cup plain yogurt

1/2 cup water or coconut water

1 tablespoon honey or maple syrup (optional)

Instructions:

In a blender, combine the frozen berries, yogurt, water, and honey.

Blend until smooth.

Pour the mixture into popsicle molds.

Insert sticks and freeze for at least 4 hours or until solid.

To remove, run warm water over the outside of the molds for a few seconds.

Cooking Time: None (freezing time: 4 hours)

37. Banana and Nut Muffins

Ingredients:

1 cup mashed ripe bananas (about 2 large bananas)

1/2 cup almond flour

1/4 cup chopped nuts (e.g., walnuts or pecans)

2 tablespoons honey or maple syrup

1/2 teaspoon baking powder

1/4 teaspoon baking soda

A pinch of salt

Instructions:

Preheat oven to 350°F (175°C) and line a muffin tin with paper liners.

In a bowl, mix together the almond flour, baking powder, baking soda, and salt.

In another bowl, combine the mashed bananas and honey.

Add the wet ingredients to the dry ingredients and mix until just combined.

Fold in the chopped nuts.

Spoon the batter into the muffin tin, filling each cup about 2/3 full.

Bake for 15-18 minutes, or until a toothpick inserted into the center comes out clean.

Let muffins cool in the tin for 5 minutes before transferring to a wire rack to cool completely.

Cooking Time: 15-18 minutes

38. Homemade Soft Granola Bars

Ingredients:

1 cup rolled oats

1/2 cup almond butter

1/4 cup honey or maple syrup

1/4 cup dried fruit (e.g., raisins or cranberries)

1/4 cup chopped nuts or seeds (optional)

Instructions:

Line an 8x8-inch baking dish with parchment paper.

In a saucepan, heat the almond butter and honey over low heat until melted and well combined.

In a bowl, mix the oats, dried fruit, and nuts or seeds.

Pour the almond butter mixture over the dry ingredients and stir until evenly coated.

Press the mixture firmly into the prepared dish.

Refrigerate for at least 2 hours to set.

Once set, cut into bars and store in an airtight container.

Cooking Time: None (chilling time: 2 hours)

39. Cucumber and Turkey Roll-Ups

Ingredients:

1 large cucumber

4 slices turkey breast (deli or cooked)

2 tablespoons cream cheese or hummus

A pinch of salt and pepper (optional)

Instructions:

Peel the cucumber and slice it lengthwise into thin strips.

Spread cream cheese or hummus on each turkey slice.

Roll each turkey slice around a cucumber strip.

Secure with a toothpick if needed.

Serve immediately or refrigerate until ready to eat.

Cooking Time: None (prep time: 5 minutes)

40. Baked Sweet Potato Chips

Ingredients:

2 medium sweet potatoes

1 tablespoon olive oil

A pinch of salt

A pinch of paprika or cinnamon (optional)

Instructions:

Preheat oven to 400°F (200°C) and line a baking sheet with parchment paper.

Peel and thinly slice the sweet potatoes using a mandolin or sharp knife.

Toss the sweet potato slices with olive oil, salt, and optional spices.

Arrange slices in a single layer on the baking sheet.

Bake for 20-25 minutes, flipping halfway through, until crispy and golden brown.

Allow chips to cool before serving.

Cooking Time: 20-25 minutes

41. Baked Apples with Cinnamon

Ingredients:

4 medium apples (such as Gala or Fuji)

2 tablespoons honey or maple syrup

1 teaspoon ground cinnamon

1/4 teaspoon ground nutmeg

2 tablespoons raisins (optional)

1/4 cup water

Instructions:

Preheat your oven to 350°F (175°C).

Core the apples, creating a hollow center. Place them in a baking dish.

In a small bowl, mix honey, cinnamon, nutmeg, and raisins (if using). Spoon this mixture into the center of each apple.

Pour water into the bottom of the baking dish.

Cover with foil and bake for 25-30 minutes, or until the apples are tender but still hold their shape.

Remove from oven and let cool slightly before serving.

Cooking Time: 25-30 minutes

42. Coconut Milk Rice Pudding

Ingredients:

1/2 cup short-grain rice

2 cups coconut milk

1/4 cup honey or maple syrup

1/2 teaspoon vanilla extract

Pinch of salt

Instructions:

Rinse the rice under cold water.

In a medium saucepan, combine rice, coconut milk, honey, vanilla, and salt.

Bring to a boil over medium heat, then reduce to low and cover.

Simmer for 25-30 minutes, stirring occasionally, until the rice is tender and the pudding has thickened.

Let cool slightly before serving.

Cooking Time: 25-30 minutes

43. Soft-Baked Pear Muffins

Ingredients:

1 1/2 cups whole wheat flour

1/2 cup oat flour

1/2 cup honey

1/2 cup unsweetened applesauce

1/2 cup finely diced ripe pears

1/4 cup olive oil

2 large eggs

1 teaspoon baking powder

1/2 teaspoon baking soda

1/2 teaspoon ground cinnamon

Instructions:

Preheat your oven to 350°F (175°C). Line a muffin tin with paper liners.

In a large bowl, whisk together flour, oat flour, baking powder, baking soda, and cinnamon.

In another bowl, mix honey, applesauce, olive oil, and eggs.

Add wet ingredients to dry ingredients and stir until just combined. Gently fold in diced pears.

Divide batter evenly among muffin cups.

Bake for 20-25 minutes, or until a toothpick inserted into the center comes out clean.

Cool in the pan for 5 minutes, then transfer to a wire rack to cool completely.

Cooking Time: 20-25 minutes

44. Vanilla Chia Seed Pudding

Ingredients:

1/4 cup chia seeds

1 cup almond milk (or other non-dairy milk)

2 tablespoons honey or maple syrup

1/2 teaspoon vanilla extract

Instructions:

In a bowl, combine chia seeds, almond milk, honey, and vanilla extract.

Stir well and let sit for 10 minutes. Stir again to prevent clumping.

Cover and refrigerate for at least 2 hours, or overnight, until the pudding has thickened.

Stir before serving.

Cooking Time: 10 minutes (plus chilling time)

45. Banana Oat Cookies

Ingredients:

2 ripe bananas

1 cup rolled oats

1/4 cup raisins (optional)

1/2 teaspoon ground cinnamon

Instructions:

Preheat your oven to 350°F (175°C). Line a baking sheet with parchment paper.

In a bowl, mash the bananas until smooth.

Stir in oats, raisins (if using), and cinnamon.

Drop spoonfuls of the mixture onto the prepared baking sheet, flattening them slightly.

Bake for 10-12 minutes, or until cookies are golden brown.

Cool on a wire rack before serving.

Cooking Time: 10-12 minutes

46. Berry Compote with Yogurt

Ingredients:

2 cups mixed berries (fresh or frozen)

1/4 cup honey or maple syrup

1 tablespoon lemon juice

1 cup plain Greek yogurt (or a dairy-free alternative)

Instructions:

In a saucepan, combine berries, honey, and lemon juice.

Cook over medium heat, stirring occasionally, for 10-15 minutes, or until berries break down and the mixture thickens.

Let cool slightly.

Serve a spoonful of compote over Greek yogurt.

Cooking Time: 10-15 minutes

47. Simple Apple Sauce

Ingredients:

4 medium apples, peeled, cored, and chopped

1/4 cup water

2 tablespoons honey or maple syrup (optional)

1/2 teaspoon ground cinnamon (optional)

Instructions:

In a saucepan, combine apples and water.

Cover and cook over medium heat for 15-20 minutes, or until apples are soft.

Mash apples with a fork or blend with an immersion blender until smooth.

Stir in honey and cinnamon, if using.

Let cool before serving.

Cooking Time: 15-20 minutes

48. Pumpkin Custard

Ingredients:

1 cup canned pumpkin puree

1/2 cup coconut milk

1/4 cup honey or maple syrup

2 large eggs

1/2 teaspoon ground cinnamon

1/4 teaspoon ground nutmeg

Pinch of salt

Instructions:

Preheat your oven to 350°F (175°C).

In a bowl, whisk together pumpkin puree, coconut milk, honey, eggs, cinnamon, nutmeg, and salt.

Pour the mixture into ramekins or a baking dish.

Place the ramekins in a baking dish filled with hot water (about halfway up the sides of the ramekins).

Bake for 30-35 minutes, or until custard is set.

Let cool before serving.

Cooking Time: 30-35 minutes

49. Mild Mango Sorbet

Ingredients:

2 cups ripe mango chunks (fresh or frozen)

1/4 cup honey or maple syrup

1 tablespoon lime juice

Instructions:

In a blender, combine mango chunks, honey, and lime juice.

Blend until smooth.

Pour mixture into a shallow dish and freeze for 1-2 hours, stirring every 30 minutes until firm.

Scoop and serve.

Cooking Time: 1-2 hours (freezing time)

50. Pear and Ginger Compote

Ingredients:

4 ripe pears, peeled, cored, and diced

1 tablespoon fresh ginger, grated

1/4 cup honey or maple syrup

1/4 cup water

Instructions:

In a saucepan, combine pears, ginger, honey, and water.

Cook over medium heat, stirring occasionally, for 15-20 minutes, or until pears are tender and the mixture has thickened.

Let cool slightly before serving.

Cooking Time: 15-20 minutes

Day 1:

Breakfast: Creamy Oatmeal with Banana

Lunch: Chicken and Carrot Stew

Snack: Apple Slices with Almond Butter

Dinner: Baked Salmon with Dill Sauce and Steamed Rice

Dessert: Baked Apples with Cinnamon

Day 2:

Breakfast: Smoothie with Blueberries and Yogurt

Lunch: Quinoa Salad with Cucumbers and Herbs

Snack: Carrot Sticks with Hummus

Dinner: Turkey and Sweet Potato Skillet

Dessert: Coconut Milk Rice Pudding

Day 3:

Breakfast: Pumpkin Spice Chia Pudding

Lunch: Simple Chicken and Rice Soup

Snack: Rice Cakes with Avocado

Dinner: Baked Chicken Breast with Herbs and Steamed Broccoli

Dessert: Vanilla Chia Seed Pudding

Day 4:

Breakfast: Overnight Oats with Almond Milk

Lunch: Sweet Potato and Leek Soup

Snack: Yogurt with Honey and Blueberries

Dinner: Stuffed Bell Peppers with Rice

Dessert: Berry Compote with Yogurt

Day 5:

Breakfast: Soft-Baked Sweet Potato Hash

Lunch: Carrot and Ginger Soup

Snack: Smoothie Popsicles

Dinner: Steamed Fish with Lemon and Dill, served with Quinoa

Dessert: Banana Oat Cookies

Day 6:

Breakfast: Scrambled Eggs with Spinach

Lunch: Pureed Cauliflower Soup

Snack: Banana and Nut Muffins

Dinner: Chicken and Carrot Stew (leftovers) with a side of Steamed Green Beans

Dessert: Soft-Baked Pear Muffins

Day 7:

Breakfast: Cottage Cheese and Berries Parfait

Lunch: Mild Tomato Soup

Snack: Homemade Soft Granola Bars

Dinner: Soft-Cooked Pasta with Olive Oil and Herbs and a side of Steamed Zucchini

Dessert: Pear and Ginger Compote

This meal plan is designed to be gentle on the digestive system while providing balanced nutrition.

Each meal includes easy-to-digest ingredients and avoids common irritants, aiming to support overall well-being.

Chapter 8: Special Considerations

Managing Flare-Ups with Diet

Recognizing and responding to Symptoms

Ulcerative colitis manifests in a range of symptoms that can vary in intensity, making it crucial to stay vigilant.

Key signs include abdominal pain, frequent diarrhea, and rectal bleeding. Identifying these symptoms early can help manage flare-ups effectively and maintain a higher quality of life.

When symptoms appear, it's important to document their frequency, duration, and any potential triggers.

This helps in understanding patterns and making informed dietary adjustments. For instance, if certain foods seem to exacerbate symptoms, eliminating or modifying them can be beneficial.

Immediate responses include opting for easily digestible foods and staying hydrated.

Simple, bland meals can ease digestive stress, while clear broths and herbal teas can soothe the gut. During flare-ups, it's also essential to avoid high-fiber and spicy foods, which might worsen symptoms.

Regular consultation with healthcare professionals complements dietary changes, ensuring a comprehensive approach to managing ulcerative colitis.

By recognizing symptoms promptly and responding with targeted dietary strategies, you can better control your condition and improve your overall well-being.

This cookbook provides practical, tailored recipes to support you through these challenges, making your journey with ulcerative colitis smoother and more manageable.

Adjusting Diet during Flare-Ups

During flare-ups, the right diet becomes crucial for managing symptoms and promoting healing. When ulcerative colitis flares, your digestive system becomes more sensitive, and certain foods can exacerbate discomfort.

It's essential to focus on meals that are easy to digest and minimize inflammation.

Opt for bland, low-fiber foods such as plain rice, well-cooked carrots, and mashed potatoes. These options are gentle on the stomach and can help reduce irritation.

Avoid high-fiber foods, dairy products, and spicy or greasy foods, as they can trigger or worsen symptoms.

Incorporate soothing broths and clear soups to keep hydrated and provide essential nutrients without taxing your digestive system. Cooked fruits and vegetables, such as applesauce or steamed zucchini, offer vitamins while being gentle on the gut.

Pay attention to portion sizes and eat smaller, more frequent meals to avoid overwhelming your digestive system.

Keeping a food diary can help identify which foods contribute to flare-ups, allowing for more personalized dietary adjustments.

By tailoring your diet during flare-ups, you can alleviate discomfort and support your body's healing process, paving the way for better management of ulcerative colitis.

Identifying and Avoiding Trigger Foods

Common Trigger Foods

Living with ulcerative colitis requires careful attention to diet, as certain foods can exacerbate symptoms and lead to discomfort.

Identifying and avoiding these trigger foods is essential for managing your condition effectively.

Certain high-fiber foods, such as raw vegetables, nuts, and whole grains, can be difficult to digest and may irritate the digestive tract. Dairy products often pose a challenge, as they can cause bloating and diarrhea due to lactose intolerance, which is prevalent among individuals with ulcerative colitis.

Spicy foods and caffeine are known to stimulate the gut, potentially leading to increased symptoms.

Fatty and fried foods are another category to watch out for, as they can be hard on your system and may trigger flare-ups.

Additionally, artificial sweeteners and high-sugar foods can disrupt gut health and contribute to inflammation.

Understanding your personal triggers involves paying close attention to how your body responds to different foods.

By eliminating or modifying these problem foods, you can find relief and improve your overall well-being.

This cookbook provides recipes that prioritize gentle, healing ingredients to help you maintain a balanced diet while managing ulcerative colitis.

How to Determine Personal Triggers

Understanding your unique food triggers is crucial for managing ulcerative colitis effectively.

Each person's digestive system reacts differently, so identifying what exacerbates your symptoms involves a thoughtful and systematic approach.

Start by keeping a detailed food diary. Record everything you eat and drink, including portion sizes and meal times. Alongside your dietary notes, track your symptoms—both the intensity and timing.

This detailed log will help you spot patterns and identify potential triggers.

Next, consider eliminating suspected problem foods from your diet one at a time.

Common culprits include high-fiber foods, dairy products, and spicy dishes. Reintroduce these foods gradually, observing any changes in your symptoms. This process can help pinpoint which foods may be causing issues.

Consulting with a healthcare professional or dietitian can also be beneficial.

They can provide personalized advice based on your food diary and help you adjust your diet to avoid triggers while ensuring balanced nutrition.

By methodically tracking and testing your food intake, you can gain a clearer understanding of your personal triggers and make informed choices to manage your ulcerative colitis effectively.

Nutritional Supplements and Ulcerative Colitis

Essential Nutrients and Supplements

Managing ulcerative colitis requires more than just careful meal planning; it also involves ensuring you get the right nutrients to support your overall health. Essential nutrients play a crucial role in maintaining your body's strength and aiding in recovery.

For individuals with ulcerative colitis, focusing on a balanced intake of vitamins and minerals is vital.

Fiber is key for digestive health, but it should be introduced gradually and in moderation to avoid aggravating symptoms.

Omega-3 fatty acids, found in fish oil, can help reduce inflammation and promote gut health.

Vitamin D is important for immune function and bone health, especially if you're on medications that affect bone density.

Probiotics can support a healthy gut microbiome, potentially alleviating symptoms and improving digestion.

In some cases, supplements like calcium and iron may be necessary, especially if your condition affects nutrient absorption or if you're on a restricted diet.

Always consult with a healthcare provider before starting any supplements to ensure they're appropriate for your specific needs.

Incorporating these essential nutrients and supplements into your routine can provide significant benefits, complementing the healing power of your diet and supporting your journey to better health.

Consulting with a Healthcare Provider

When managing ulcerative colitis, consulting with a healthcare provider is a crucial step toward achieving optimal health.

Your provider is your partner in understanding the complexities of your condition and tailoring a treatment plan that suits your unique needs. They offer valuable insights into how dietary changes can complement your overall treatment strategy.

Regular consultations allow you to discuss symptoms, track progress, and adjust your diet as needed.

A healthcare provider can help identify which foods may trigger flare-ups and offer guidance on nutritional needs specific to ulcerative colitis.

Their expertise ensures that you are making informed choices that support your well-being without compromising on nutrition.

Engaging with a healthcare provider also means you have a support system in place for managing medication and understanding any potential interactions with dietary changes.

They can help you stay on top of your condition and adapt your approach as needed, making your journey toward better health more manageable and effective. Prioritizing these consultations is an essential part of living well with ulcerative colitis and making the most of the dietary strategies outlined in this cookbook.

Benefits of following the Diet

Short-Term and Long-Term Health Benefits

Following a tailored diet designed for ulcerative colitis can lead to significant improvements in both the short term and long term. In the short term, carefully selected recipes can help alleviate immediate symptoms, such as abdominal pain and discomfort.

Meals crafted with anti-inflammatory ingredients and gentle, easy-to-digest components can soothe the digestive tract, reducing flare-ups and enhancing overall comfort. By focusing on gut-friendly foods, individuals can experience quicker relief from symptoms and improved digestion.

Over time, adhering to a specialized diet can foster more profound, long-lasting health benefits.

Consistent, balanced meals support the healing of the intestinal lining and help maintain remission, reducing the frequency and severity of flare-ups.

A diet rich in essential nutrients strengthens the immune system and promotes overall wellness, contributing to better quality of life. Long-term adherence to a carefully crafted diet can also minimize the need for medication and reduce healthcare costs by preventing complications and hospital visits.

The Complete Ulcerative Colitis Cookbook offers a pathway to both immediate relief and sustained well-being, empowering individuals to take control of their health through thoughtful, nourishing meals.

Improving Quality of Life

Living with ulcerative colitis often means facing daily challenges that impact your overall well-being. But by embracing a diet tailored to manage symptoms, you can significantly enhance your quality of life.

This cookbook offers more than just recipes; it provides a pathway to feeling better and regaining control.

Each meal plan is crafted to be gentle on the digestive system while delivering essential nutrients.

By focusing on easy-to-digest, anti-inflammatory foods, you reduce the risk of flare-ups and support your body's healing process.

Simple changes in your diet can lead to fewer disruptions, improved energy levels, and a more stable mood.

Imagine a day where meal times no longer bring anxiety, but instead offer comfort and satisfaction. With carefully selected ingredients and recipes designed to fit your needs, this cookbook helps turn that vision into reality. By following these meal plans, you're not just managing symptoms—you're investing in a healthier, more enjoyable life.

Embrace this approach and discover how nourishing your body with the right foods can lead to a more balanced and fulfilling life.

Conclusion

As we reach the end of The Complete Ulcerative Colitis Cookbook, it's important to reflect on the journey you've embarked upon and the transformation that's possible through thoughtful dietary choices.

This book has been designed to offer more than just recipes; it is a guide to improving your quality of life, managing symptoms, and finding joy in the food you eat.

Living with ulcerative colitis requires a nuanced approach to diet, and the recipes within these pages are crafted with your well-being in mind.

By incorporating these meal plans into your routine, you're not just avoiding discomfort—you're nurturing your body with nutrients that support healing and balance.

Remember, the path to managing ulcerative colitis is a personal one, and while this cookbook provides a foundation, it's essential to adapt and modify recipes to suit your unique needs. Listening to your body and working closely with your healthcare team will help you tailor these suggestions to what works best for you.

Thank you for allowing this book to be a part of your journey.

May these recipes bring comfort, satisfaction, and a renewed sense of control over your health. Here's to a future filled with nourishing meals and a life lived with greater ease and joy.

Dear Readers,

Thank you for choosing The Complete Ulcerative Colitis Cookbook as your companion on this journey to better health and wellness.

It has been my honor to share these recipes and insights with you, and I hope they bring comfort, nourishment, and a renewed sense of enjoyment to your meals.

Your feedback is incredibly valuable, and I would love to hear about your experiences with the recipes and how this book has impacted your life. If you found this cookbook helpful, please consider leaving a review and rating.

Your thoughts not only help others discover this resource but also allow me to continue improving and supporting the community.

Thank you once again for your trust and support. Wishing you many happy, healthy meals and a future filled with vibrant health.

Warm regards,

[Nancy Rios]

www.ingramcontent.com/pod-product-compliance
Lightning Source LLC
Chambersburg PA
CBHW071040250726
48653CB00005B/1930